THE APPLICATION OF COMPARATIVE MORPHOLOGY IN THE IDENTIFICATION OF INTESTINAL PARASITES

Publication Number 908

AMERICAN LECTURE SERIES

A Publication in

The BANNERSTONE DIVISION *of*
AMERICAN LECTURES IN CLINICAL MICROBIOLOGY

Edited by

ALBERT BALOWS, Ph.D.

Chief, Bacteriology Branch
Center for Disease Control
Atlanta, Georgia   30322

THE APPLICATION OF COMPARATIVE MORPHOLOGY IN THE IDENTIFICATION OF INTESTINAL PARASITES

$\left[\ \text{In Full Color}\ \right]$

By

JOHN W. MOOSE, M.S., LTC, A.U.S. (Ret.)

Parasitology Section
Division of Personal
Health Laboratories
Bureau of Laboratories
South Carolina State Board of Health
Columbia, South Carolina

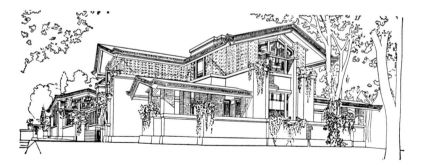

CHARLES C THOMAS • PUBLISHER
Springfield • Illinois • U.S.A.

Published and Distributed Throughout the World by

CHARLES C THOMAS • PUBLISHER

Bannerstone House

301-327 East Lawrence Avenue, Springfield, Illinois, U.S.A.

©*1973, by* CHARLES C THOMAS • PUBLISHER

ISBN 0-398-02874-5

Library of Congress Catalog Card Number: 73-5867

*With THOMAS BOOKS careful attention is given to all details of
manufacturing and design. It is the Publisher's desire to present books that
are satisfactory as to their physical qualities and artistic possibilities and
appropriate for their particular use. THOMAS BOOKS will be true to those
laws of quality that assure a good name and good will.*

Printed in the United States of America

R-1

This book is dedicated to the memory of my late father, Colonel Frank McA. Moose, M.C., U.S.A. (Ret.), who devoted his life to the welfare of his patients.

FOREWORD

THE genesis of this series, *The American Lecture Series in Clinical Microbiology,* stems from the concerted efforts of the Editor and the Publisher to provide a forum from which well-qualified and distinguished authors may present, either as a book or monograph, their views on any aspect of clinical microbiology. Our definition of clinical microbiology is conceived to encompass the broadest aspects of medical microbiology not only as it is applied to the clinical laboratory but equally to the research laboratory and to theoretical considerations. In the clinical microbiology laboratory we are concerned with differences in morphology, biochemical behavior and antigenic patterns as a means of microbial identification. In the research laboratory or when we employ microorganisms as a model in theoretical biology, our interest is often focused not so much on the above differences but rather on the similarities between microorganisms. However, it must be appreciated that even though there are many similarities between cells, there are important differences between major types of cells which set very definite limits on the cellular behavior. Unless this is understood it is impossible to discern common denominators.

We are also concerned with the relationships between micro-organism and disease – any microorganism and any disease. Implicit in these relations is the role of the host which forms the third arm of the triangle: microorganism, disease and host. In this series we plan to explore each of these; singly where possible for factual information and in combination for an understanding of the myriad of interrelationships that exist. This necessitates the application of basic principles of biology and may, at times, require the emergence of new theoretical concepts which will create new principles or modify existing ones. Above all, our aim is to present well-documented books which will be informative, instructive and useful, creating a sense of satisfaction to both the reader and the author.

Closely intertwined with the above *raison d'être* is our desire to produce a series which will be read not only for the pleasure of knowledge but which will also enhance the reader's professional skill and extend his technical ability. *The American Lecture Series in Clinical Microbiology* is dedicated to biologists — be they physicians, scientists or teachers — in the hope that this series will foster better appreciation of mutual problems and help close the gap between theoretical and applied microbiology.

Parasitology, insofar as it is performed in clinical and public health laboratories, has consistently been the most neglected discipline in clinical and diagnostic microbiology. This neglect, to a large measure, is due to inadequate training and a lack of *good* instructional material. There is also an obvious void in interpretation when inexperienced persons are confronted with actual specimens as seen under the microscope.

It is difficult for many individuals to utilize correctly information gained from chalkboard or textbook drawings or authoritative descriptions of the diagnostic stages of intestinal parasites. This addition to *The American Lecture Series in Clinical Microbiology* is a positive approach toward solving this problem. This manual is designed to impart almost immediate understanding to the bench worker and, at the same time, should be very useful as a reference in the lecture room and library of all clinical laboratory workers.

The author, Colonel John W. Moose, has had more than twenty years of experience as a parasitologist in this country and abroad. Colonel Moose was Chief of the Department of Medical Zoology of the 406th Medical Laboratory of the U.S. Army Medical Command in Japan. He was also Chief of the Parasitology Section and Microbiology Branch, Pathology and Laboratory Sciences Division, U.S. Army Medical Field Service School in Fort Sam Houston, Texas. Presently, he is parasitologist of the Bureau of Laboratories of the South Carolina State Board of Health. While serving in all of these assignments, the author has prepared an invaluable collection of colored photomicrographs of protozoan and helminth parasites. In this book, Colonel Moose has assembled 136 of those photomicrographs which accurately depict the characteristic and diagnostic features of those intestinal parasites of man most likely to be seen in the United States.

The reader of this book will observe at first glance that the narrative is held to a minimum. After all, one good picture is worth a thousand words!

ALBERT BALOWS, Ph.D.
Editor

INTRODUCTION

THIS color atlas of the diagnostic stages of intestinal parasites is intended to be used as a training aid by teachers, laboratory personnel, medical students and physicians in the recognition and identification of intestinal parasites. The manual consists of 136 color photomicrographs of actual diagnostic forms of protozoan and helminth parasites and some pseudoparasites. The majority of the parasites depicted are indigenous to the United States; however, a few do not naturally occur in this country, but may on rare occasion be seen in routine diagnostic work. These exotic organisms may be recovered in specimens from persons who acquired the infection in areas of the world where the parasite is endemic.

Although the habitats of *Clonorchis sinensis, Dicrocoelium dendriticum, Fasciola hepatica, Opisthorchis viverrini, Paragonimus westermani, Schistosoma japonicum* and *S. mansoni* are other than the lumen of the intestine, their eggs are encountered in fecal specimens. Therefore, these organisms are included with the intestinal parasites. The egg of *S. haematobium* is, of course, recovered in urine; it is included here for completeness.

The format of the manual is unique in that the sequence of the photographs, for the most part, is based on comparative morphology of the diagnostic stages rather than a taxonomic arrangement. Where feasible, organisms which resemble each other are placed close together so that the student will have a better understanding of the material presented during lecture periods and, most important, will immediately visualize the size relationship and other specific morphological similarities and/or differences between each of the organisms illustrated.

A few pseudoparasites, or objects that are often mistaken for protozoan cysts or helminth eggs and larvae, are incorporated in appropriate places.

Under each photograph the name of the organism, the diagnostic stage, the actual magnification used in photomicrography, the stain employed in preparation of the material and the more practical criteria to be used for identification of the parasites are presented.

Special mention must be made that this bench manual is intended to be complementary to various parasitology textbooks already available. Therefore, it is not the author's purpose to include narrative text material concerning the parasites nor detailed laboratory procedures. This information may be found in the textbooks listed under references.

The author is grateful to Arthur F. DiSalvo, M. D., Chief, Bureau of Laboratories, South Carolina State Board of Health, Columbia, South Carolina for his keen interest in this work and being instrumental in its ultimate publication. Appreciation is expressed to George R. Healy, Ph.D., Chief, Helminthology and Protozoology Unit and Dorothy M. Melvin, Ph.D., Chief, Parasitology Training Unit, Center for Disease Control, Atlanta, Georgia who supplied the preserved fecal specimens containing *Isospora belli* and *I. hominis* oocysts respectively for photomicrography.

Grateful acknowledgment is extended to Anne Reddick, Ph.D., Director, Division of Personal Health Laboratories, Bureau of Laboratories, South Carolina State Board of Health for her critical review of the manuscript.

CONTENTS

THE APPLICATION OF
COMPARATIVE MORPHOLOGY
IN THE IDENTIFICATION OF
INTESTINAL PARASITES

THE BENCH MANUAL

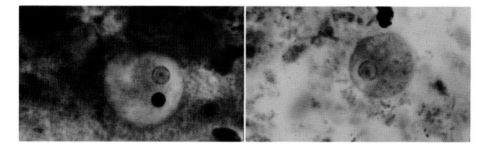

Figure 1. *Entamoeba histolytica* trophozoite, invasive form, Wheatley's trichrome stained fecal smear, X1000. Criteria: Small karyosome; clean, delicate nucleus; clean cytoplasm. Note: Dark staining ingested red blood cell in the cytoplasm.

Figure 2. *Entamoeba coli* trophozoite, Heidenhain's iron-hematoxylin stained fecal smear, X1000. Criteria: Small karyosome; dirty, coarse nucleus; dirty cytoplasm; perinuclear space. Note: Dark staining ingested bacteria in the cytoplasm. Although the perinuclear space is not present in all *E. coli* trophozoites, it occurs often enough so that it can be employed as a helpful criterion for identification.

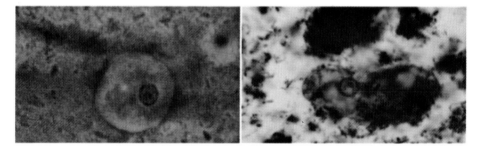

Figure 3. *Entamoeba histolytica* trophozoite, invasive form, Heidenhain's iron-hematoxylin stained fecal smear, X1000. Criteria: Small karyosome; clean, delicate nucleus; clean cytoplasm. Note: The invasive form trophozoite does not ingest bacteria.

Figure 4. *Entamoeba coli* trophozoite, Heidenhain's iron-hematoxylin stained fecal smear, X1000. Criteria: Small karyosome; dirty, coarse nucleus; dirty cytoplasm. Note: The empty vacuoles in the cytoplasm of trophozoites are due to degeneration of the organism before fixation.

5

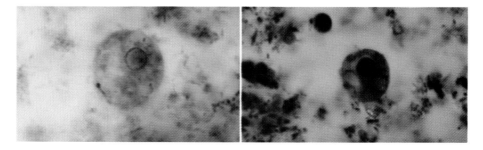

Figure 5. *Entamoeba coli* trophozoite, Heidenhain's iron-hematoxylin stained fecal smear, X1000. Criteria: Small karyosome; dirty, coarse nucleus; dirty cytoplasm.

Figure 6. *Entamoeba coli* trophozoite, Heidenhain's iron-hematoxylin stained fecal smear, X1000. Criteria: Small karyosome; dirty, coarse nucleus; dirty cytoplasm, perinuclear space.

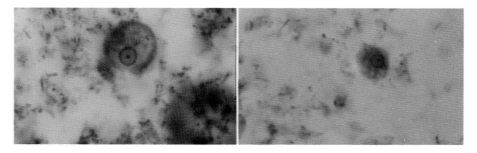

Figure 7. *Entamoeba histolytica* trophozoite, commensal form, Heidenhain's iron-hematoxylin stained fecal smear, X1000. Criteria: Small karyosome; clean, delicate nucleus; relatively clean cytoplasm. Note: The commensal form trophozoite does ingest bacteria.

Figure 8. *Entamoeba hartmanni* trophozoite, Heidenhain's iron-hematoxylin stained fecal smear, X1000. Criteria: Small karyosome; obvious small size of the organism.

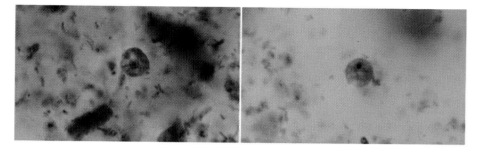

Figure 9. *Endolimax nana* trophozoite, Wheatley's trichrome stained fecal smear, X1000. Criteria: Large karyosome; well defined nuclear membrane; clear area between the karyosome and the nuclear membrane.

Figure 10. *Endolimax nana* trophozoite, Heidenhain's iron-hematoxylin stained fecal smear, X1000. Criteria: Large karyosome; well defined nuclear membrane; clear area between the karyosome and the nuclear membrane.

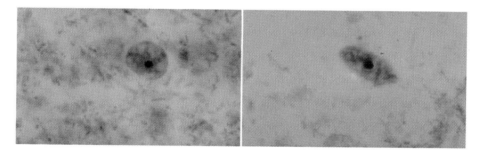

Figure 11. *Iodamoeba bütschlii* trophozoite, Heidenhain's iron-hematoxylin stained fecal smear, X1000. Criteria: Large karyosome; ill-defined nuclear membrane; small granules surrounding the karyosome. Note: The granules are difficult to see in this illustration.

Figure 12. *Iodamoeba bütschlii* trophozoite, Heidenhain's iron-hematoxylin stained fecal smear, X1000. Criteria: Large karyosome; ill-defined nuclear membrane. Note: The granules are oriented on one side of the karyosome.

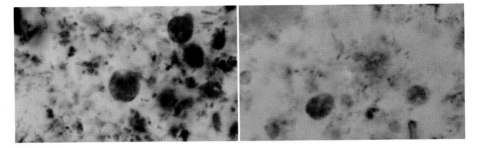

Figure 13. *Endolimax nana* trophozoites, Heidenhain's iron-hematoxylin stained fecal smear, X1000. Criteria: Large karyosome; well defined nuclear membrane; clear area between the karyosome and the nuclear membrane. Note: The outline of the karyosome is often irregular. See the organism in the center of this illustration.

Figure 14. *Endolimax nana* (left) and *Entamoeba hartmanni* (right) trophozoites, Heidenhain's iron-hematoxylin stained fecal smear, X1000. Note: Occasionally, *E. hartmanni* trophozoites are smaller than those of *E. nana*.

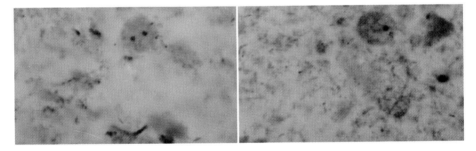

Figure 15. *Dientamoeba fragilis* trophozoite, Heidenhain's iron-hematoxylin stained fecal smear, X1000. Criteria: Fractured karyosome; two nuclei.

Figure 16. *Dientamoeba fragilis* trophozoite, Heidenhain's iron-hematoxylin stained fecal smear, X1000. Criterion: Fractured karyosome. Note: It is not unusual for this organism to possess only one nucleus.

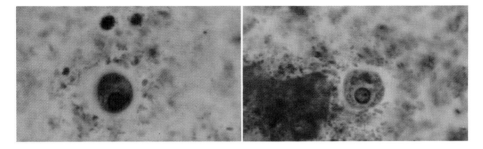

Figure 17. *Entamoeba histolytica* pre-cyst, Wheatley's trichrome stained fecal smear, X1000. Criteria: Shape usually spherical; one large nucleus. Note: Pre-cysts and especially uninucleate cysts are frequently encountered in fecal specimens from persons infected with *E. histolytica*.

Figure 18. *Entamoeba histolytica* pre-cyst, Wheatley's trichrome stained fecal smear, X1000. Criteria: Shape usually spherical; one large nucleus. Note: Pre-cysts and cysts of *E. histolytica* are occasionally seen with the karyosome eccentrically located within the nucleus.

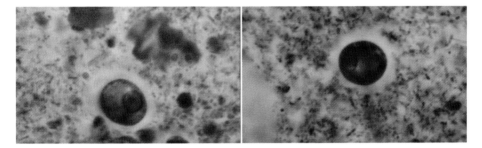

Figure 19. *Entamoeba histolytica* im-mature cyst, Wheatley's trichrome stained fecal smear, X1000. Criteria: Shape usually spherical; one large nucleus; glycogen vacuole. Note: Uninucleate cysts of *E. histolytica* are frequently observed. *E. coli* uninucleate cysts are rarely seen in a fecal specimen.

Figure 20. *Entamoeba histolytica* im-mature cyst, Heidenhain's iron-hematoxylin stained fecal smear, X1000. Criteria: Shape usually spherical; one large nucleus; multiple chromatoidal bars with rounded ends; glycogen vacuole.

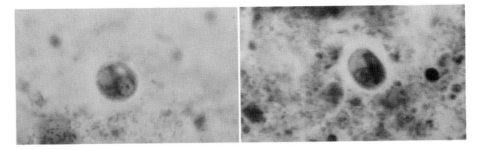

Figure 21. *Entamoeba histolytica* immature cyst, Wheatley's trichrome stained fecal smear, X1000. Criteria: Shape usually spherical; one large nucleus; cigar-shaped chromatoidal bar; glycogen vacuole.

Figure 22. *Entamoeba histolytica* immature cyst, Wheatley's trichrome stained fecal smear, X1000. Criteria: Shape usually spherical, occasionally ovoidal; one large nucleus; cigar-shaped chromatoidal bar; glycogen vacuole.

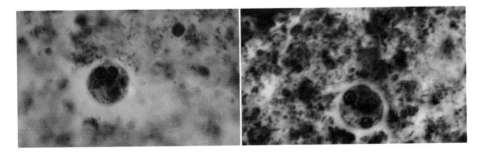

Figure 23. *Entamoeba histolytica* immature cyst, Wheatley's trichrome stained fecal smear, X1000. Criteria: Shape usually spherical; two medium sized nuclei. Note: Binucleate cysts of this species are fairly commonly seen. The nuclei are frequently located side by side.

Figure 24. *Entamoeba histolytica* immature cyst, Wheatley's trichrome stained fecal smear, X1000. Criteria: Shape usually spherical; two medium sized nuclei. Note: Occasionally, the nuclei are located at opposite poles.

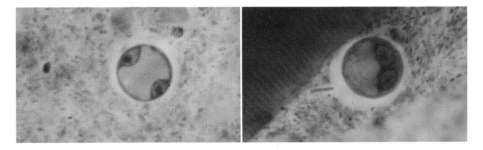

Figure 25. *Entamoeba coli* immature cyst, Heidenhain's iron-hematoxylin stained fecal smear, X1000. Criteria: Shape usually spherical; two large nuclei; glycogen vacuole. Note: Binucleate, not uninucleate, cysts of *E. coli* are commonly seen. The nuclei are frequently located at opposite poles.

Figure 26. *Entamoeba coli* immature cyst, Heidenhain's iron-hematoxylin stained fecal smear, X1000. Criteria: Shape usually spherical; two large nuclei; glycogen vacuole. Note: The nuclei may occasionally be located side by side. Notice the mitotic figure in the upper nucleus.

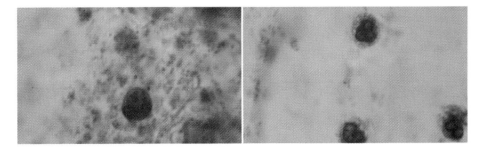

Figure 27. Segmented neutrophil, Wheatley's trichrome stained fecal smear, X1000. Criteria: Shape usually spherical; heavy, deep staining nuclear membranes; large nuclei out of proportion to the overall size of the cell. Note: These cells are often incorrectly identified as *E. histolytica* cysts.

Figure 28. Segmented neutrophilis, Wheatley's trichrome stained fecal smear, X1000. Criteria: Shapes usually spherical; heavy, deep staining nuclear membranes; large nuclei out or proportion to the overall size of the cells.

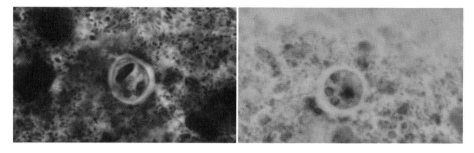

Figure 29. *Entamoeba histolytica* mature cyst, Heidenhain's iron-hematoxylin stained fecal smear, X1000. Criteria: Shape usually spherical; cigar-shaped chromatoidal bars; small nuclei. Note: Only three of four nuclei are visible in this focal plane.

Figure 30. *Entamoeba histolytica* mature cyst, Wheatley's trichrome stained fecal smear, X1000. Criteria: Shape usually spherical; small nuclei. Note: Karyosomal position is not an absolute criterion for identification of cysts belonging to this genus. The karyosome within the lower nucleus is eccentrically located while the others are more centrally positioned. The fourth nucleus is not visible in this focal plane.

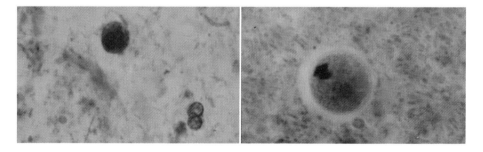

Figure 31. Segmented neutrophil, Wheatley's trichrome stained fecal smear, X1000. Criteria: Shape usually spherical; heavy, deep staining nuclear membranes; large nuclei out of proportion to the overall size of the cell.

Figure 32. *Entamoeba coli* mature cyst, Heidenhain's iron-hematoxylin stained fecal smear, X1000. Criteria: Shape usually spherical; chromatoidal bars with pointed ends. Note: All eight nuclei are not visible in this focal plane.

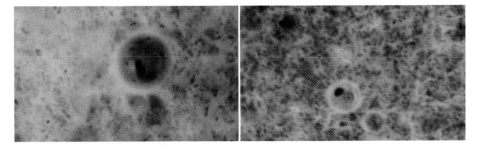

Figure 33. *Entamoeba coli* mature cyst, Heidenhain's iron-hematoxylin stained fecal smear, X1000. Criteria: Shape usually spherical; chromatoidal bars with pointed ends. Note: Only two of eight nuclei are visible in this focal plane. It is unusual for a mature cyst to contain as many chromatoidal bars as illustrated here.

Figure 34. *Entamoeba hartmanni* immature cyst, Heidenhain's iron-hematoxylin stained fecal smear, X1000. Criteria: Shape usually spherical, frequently irregular and occasionally ovoidal; obvious small size of the cyst; one large nucleus; chromatoidal bar with round ends.

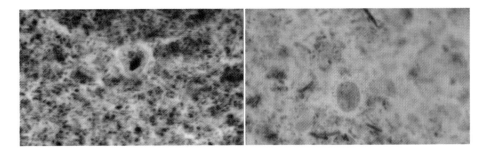

Figure 35. *Entamoeba hartmanni* immature cyst, Heidenhain's iron-hematoxylin stained fecal smear, X1000. Criteria: Shape frequently irregular, but usually spherical and sometimes ovoidal; obvious small size of the cyst; two medium sized nuclei frequently located side by side; chromatoidal bar with round ends.

Figure 36. *Endolimax nana* mature cyst, Heidenhain's iron-hematoxylin stained fecal smear, X1000. Criteria: Shape usually ovoidal, but often spherical; indefinite nuclear detail (ill-defined nuclear membranes). Note: Only two of four nuclei are visible in this focal plane.

13

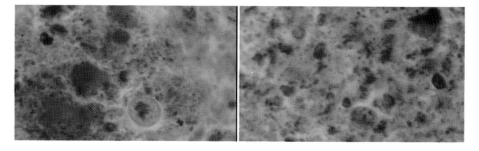

Figure 37. *Entamoeba hartmanni* mature cyst, Wheatley's trichrome stained fecal smear, X1000. Criteria: Shape usually spherical; small nuclei with well defined nuclear membranes; small, inconspicuous karyosomes. Note: Only two of four nuclei are visible in this focal plane.

Figure 38. *Endolimax nana* mature cyst, Wheatley's trichrome stained fecal smear, X1000. Criteria: Shape usually ovoidal, but may be spherical; four conspicuous karyosomes; ill-defined nuclear membranes.

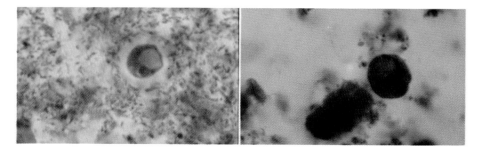

Figure 39. *Iodamoeba bütschlii* mature cyst, Heidenhain's iron-hematoxylin stained fecal smear, X1000. Criteria: Shape usually irregular, but may be spherical or ovoidal; large glycogen vacuole; large karyosome with cresent of granules usually present at one side of the karyosome; coarse cytoplasm.

Figure 40. *Iodamoeba bütschlii* mature cyst, Wheatley's trichrome stained fecal smear, X1000. Criteria: Shape spherical, but usually irregular and occasionally ovoidal; large glycogen vacuole; large karyosome with cresent of granules usually present at one side of the karyosome; coarse cytoplasm.

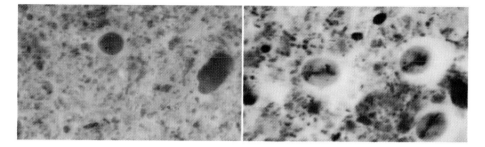

Figure 41. *Chilomastix mesnili* cyst, Wheatley's trichrome stained fecal smear, X1000. Criteria: Lemon-shaped; anterior hyaline knob; usually a well defined nucleus; light staining fibrils.

Figure 42. *Giardia lamblia* cysts, Heidenhain's iron-hematoxylin stained fecal smear, X1000. Criteria: Shapes usually ovoidal, occasionally spherical; deep staining fibrils; nuclei usually located at one end.

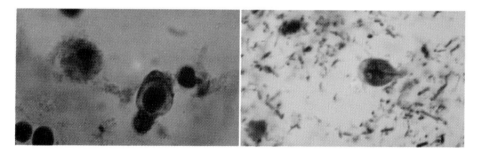

Figure 43. *Giardia lamblia* cyst ingested by a segmented neutrophil, Wheatley's trichrome stained fecal smear, X1000. Note: Our body defenses at work.

Figure 44. *Giardia lamblia* trophozoite, Heidenhain's iron-hematoxylin stained fecal smear, X1000. Criteria: Pear-shaped; two well defined nuclei; deep staining axonemes; anterior non-staining sucking disk.

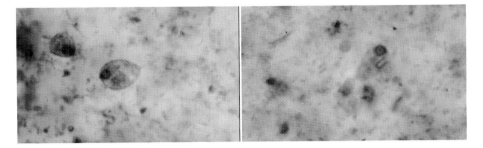

Figure 45. *Chilomastix mesnili* trophozoite, Heidenhain's iron-hematoxylin
stained fecal smear, X1000. Criteria:
Tear-shaped; nucleus touching the cell
membrane.

Figure 46. *Chilomastix mesnili* trophozoite, Heidenhain's iron-hematoxylin
stained fecal smear, X1000. Criteria:
Tear-shaped; nucleus touching the cell
membrane; conspicuous cytostome in the
immediate vicinity of the nucleus.

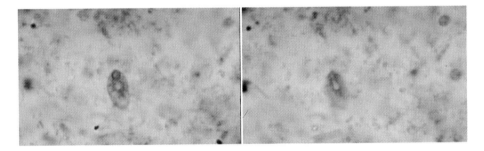

Figure 47. *Chilomastix mesnili* trophozoite, Heidenhain's iron-hematoxylin
stained fecal smear, X1000. Criteria:
Tear-shaped; nucleus touching the cell
membrane; cytostome in the immediate
vicinity of the nucleus.

Figure 48. *Chilomastix mesnili* trophozoite, Heidenhain's iron-hematoxylin
stained fecal smear, X1000. Criterion:
Conspicuous cytostome. This is the same
organism that is illustrated in Figure 47.
The photomicrograph was taken in a
different focal plane.

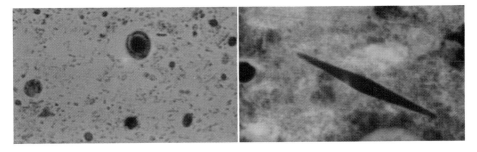

Figure 49. *Blastocystis hominis,*
Wheatley's trichrome stained fecal smear,
X1000. Criteria: Shape usually spherical;
dark staining central mass; dark staining
nuclei near the periphery of the cell.

Figure 50. Charcot-Leyden crystal,
Wheatley's trichrome stained fecal smear,
X1000. Criteria: Slender; needlelike;
sharply pointed ends. Note: These
crystals are frequently associated with
ulcerative intestinal lesions.

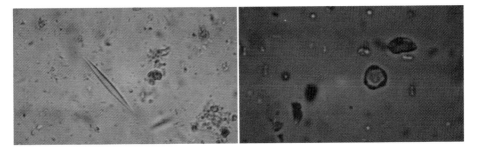

Figure 51. Charcot-Leyden crystal,
iodine stained wet fecal preparation,
X400. Criteria: Slender; needlelike;
sharply pointed ends.

Figure 52. *Blastocystis hominis,* iodine
stained wet fecal preparation, X600.
Criteria: Shape usually spherical; light
staining central mass; refractile nuclei on
the periphery of the cell.

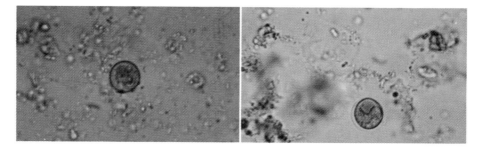

Figure 53. *Entamoeba histolytica* immature cyst, iodine stained wet fecal preparation, X600. Criteria: Shape usually spherical; one large nucleus; usually a brown glycogen mass. Note: Uninucleate cysts are frequently encountered in fecal specimens from persons infected with *E. histolytica*.

Figure 54. *Entamoeba histolytica* immature cyst, iodine stained wet fecal preparation, X600. Criteria: Shape usually spherical; one large nucleus; usually a brown glycogen mass.

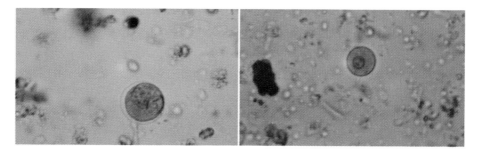

Figure 55. *Entamoeba coli* immature cyst, iodine stained wet fecal preparation, X600. Criteria: Shape usually spherical; large size of the cyst; large nucleus with coarse chromatin on the nuclear membrane; large size of the karyosome; brown glycogen mass. Note: Uninucleate cysts of *E. coli* are rarely seen in a fecal specimen. Compare the morphology of this cyst with those illustrated in Figures 53, 54 and 56.

Figure 56. *Entamoeba histolytica* immature cyst, iodine stained wet fecal preparation, X600. Criteria: Shape usually spherical; one large nucleus. Note: Because of the coarse chromatin on the nuclear membrane, this cyst could easily be mistaken for a cyst of *E. coli*. It was recovered from a fecal specimen containing many *E. histolytica* cysts. No *E. coli* cysts were observed.

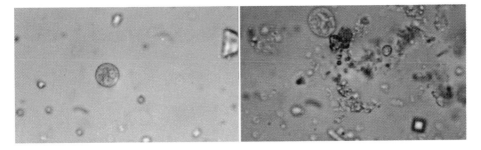

Figure 57. *Entamoeba histolytica* immature cyst, iodine stained wet fecal preparation, X600. Criteria: Shape usually spherical; chromatoidal bars with rounded ends.

Figure 58. *Entamoeba histolytica* immature cyst, unstained wet fecal preparation, X600. Criteria: Shape usually spherical; chromatoidal bars with rounded ends. Note: The contours of the bars are usually more distinct without using iodine stain.

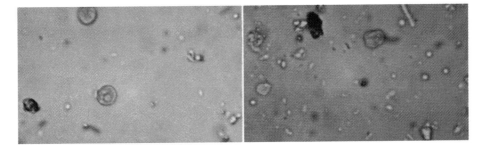

Figure 59. *Entamoeba hartmanni* immature cyst, iodine stained wet fecal preparation, X600. Criteria: Shape usually spherical, frequently irregular and occasionally ovoidal; obvious small size of the cyst; one large nucleus; chromatoidal bars with rounded ends.

Figure 60. *Entamoeba hartmanni* immature cyst, iodine stained wet fecal preparation, X600. Criteria: Shape frequently irregular, but usually spherical and sometimes ovoidal; obvious small size of the cyst; one large nucleus; chromatoidal bars with rounded ends.

19

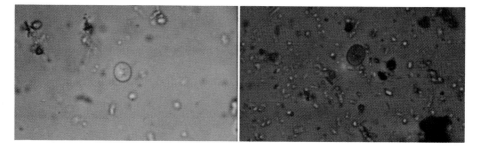

Figure 61. *Entamoeba hartmanni* mature cyst, iodine stained wet fecal preparation, X600. Criteria: Shape usually spherical; obvious small size of the cyst; nuclei with well defined nuclear membranes. Note: The fourth nucleus is not distinct in this focal plane.

Figure 62. *Endolimax nana* mature cyst, iodine stained wet fecal preparation, X600. Criteria: Shape usually ovoidal, but may be spherical; solid, refractile karyosomes, absence of nuclear membranes. Note: The fourth karyosome is not visible in this focal plane.

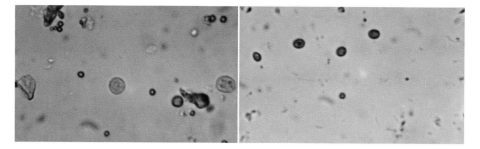

Figure 63. *Endolimax nana* mature cysts, iodine stained wet fecal preparation, X600. Criteria: Shape often spherical, but usually ovoidal; solid, refractile karyosomes; absence of nuclear membranes.

Figure 64. Small yeast cells, iodine stained wet fecal preparation, X600. Criteria: Shape usually ovoidal; intense brownish color when stained with iodine; internal structure difficult to define.

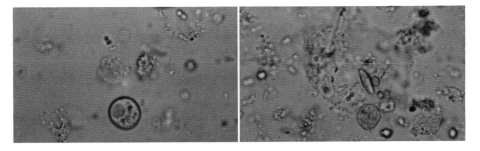

Figure 65. *Entamoeba histolytica* immature cyst, iodine stained wet fecal preparation, X600. Criteria: Shape usually spherical; two medium sized nuclei; brown glycogen mass. Note: Binucleate cysts of this species are fairly commonly seen. The nuclei are frequently located side by side.

Figure 66. *Entamoeba histolytica* immature cyst, iodine stained wet fecal preparation, X600. Criteria: Shape usually spherical; two medium sized nuclei. Note: Occasionally, the nuclei are located at opposite poles. The cyst illustrated here is rather degenerate.

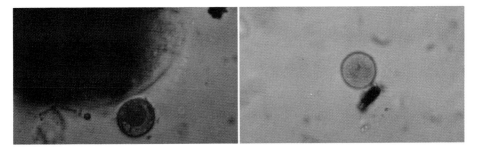

Figure 67. *Entamoeba coli* immature cyst, iodine stained wet fecal preparation, X600. Criteria: Shape usually spherical; two large nuclei; brown glycogen mass. Note: Binucleate, not uninucleate, cysts of *E. coli* are commonly seen. The nuclei are frequently located at opposite poles.

Figure 68. *Entamoeba coli* immature cyst, iodine stained wet fecal preparation, X600. Criteria: Shape usually spherical; two large nuclei. Note: The nuclei may occasionally be located side by side.

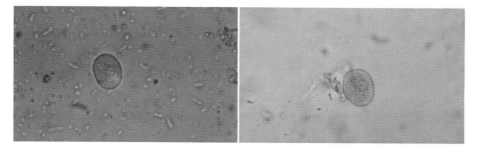

Figure 69. *Entamoeba histolytica* mature cyst, iodine stained wet fecal preparation, X600. Criteria: Shape usually spherical, occasionally ovoidal; four small nuclei.

Figure 70. *Entamoeba coli* immature cyst, iodine stained wet fecal preparation, X600. Criteria: Shape usually spherical; four large nuclei. Note: *E. coli* cysts containing four nuclei are not uncommonly seen. It is important to determine the size of the nuclei as compared to the overall size of the cyst before making an identification of *E. histolytica*.

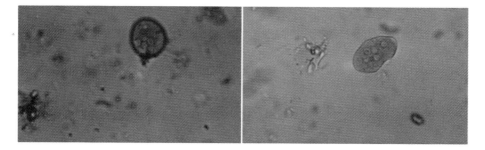

Figure 71. *Entamoeba coli* mature cyst, iodine stained wet fecal preparation, X600. Criteria: Shape usually spherical; more than four small nuclei. Note: All eight nuclei are not visible in this focal plane.

Figure 72. *Entamoeba coli* mature cyst, iodine stained wet fecal preparation, X600. Criteria: Bizarre shape; more than four small nuclei. Note: *E. coli* cysts are usually spherical; however, they may also be ovoidal, triangular or even other shapes.

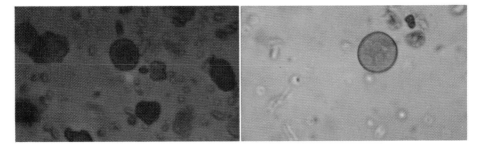

Figure 73. *Entamoeba histolytica* mature cyst, iodine stained wet fecal preparation, X600. Criteria: Shape usually spherical; four small nuclei.

Figure 74. *Entamoeba coli* immature cyst, iodine stained wet fecal preparation, X600. Criteria: Shape usually spherical; four large nuclei. Note: *E. coli* cysts containing four nuclei are not uncommonly seen. It is important to determine the size of the nuclei as compared to the overall size of the cyst before making an identification of *E. histolytica*.

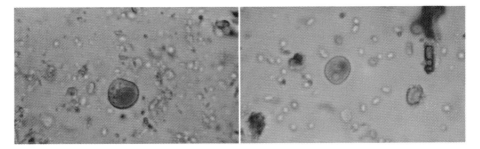

Figure 75. *Iodamoeba bütschlii* mature cyst, iodine stained wet fecal preparation, X600. Criteria: Shape usually irregular, but may be spherical or ovoidal; brown glycogen mass, coarse cytoplasm. Note: The large, refractile karyosome is not well defined in this focal plane.

Figure 76. *Iodamoeba bütschlii* mature cyst, iodine stained wet fecal preparation, X600. Criteria: Shape spherical, but usually irregular and occasionally ovoidal; brown glycogen mass; large, refractile karyosome; coarse cytoplasm.

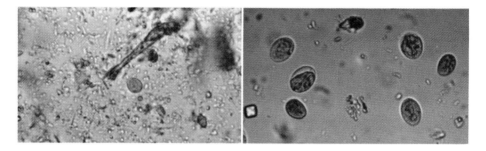

Figure 77. *Chilomastix mesnili* cyst, iodine stained wet fecal preparation, X600. Criteria: Lemon-shaped; anterior hyaline knob; usually a well defined nucleus; light staining fibrils. Note: Nuclear detail is indistinct in this focal plane.

Figure 78. *Giardia lamblia* cysts, iodine stained wet fecal preparation, X600. Criteria: Shapes usually ovoidal, occasionally spherical; deep staining fibrils; cytoplasm often retracted from the cyst wall.

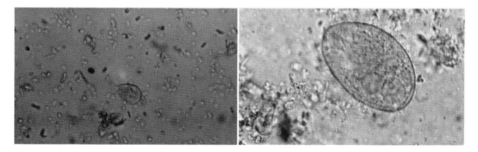

Figure 79. *Giardia lamblia* trophozoite, iodine stained wet fecal preparation, X600. Criteria: Pear-shaped; two well defined nuclei; anterior non-staining sucking disk.

Figure 80. *Balantidium coli* trophozoite, unstained wet fecal preparation, X400. Criteria: Shape ovoidal; very large size; organism covered with cilia; large contractile vacuoles usually present in the cytoplasm.

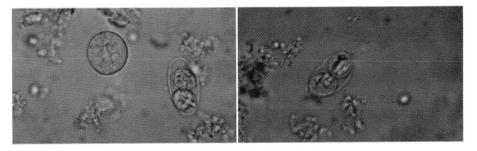

Figure 81. *Isospora hominis* immature oocyst, unstained wet fecal preparation, X600. Criteria: Shape ellipsoidal; hyaline; two sporocysts. Note: The size of the oocyst is slightly larger than the *E. coli* cyst that is also seen in this illustration.

Figure 82. *Isospora hominis* mature oocyst, unstained wet fecal preparation, X600. Criteria: Shape ellipsoidal; hyaline; two sporocysts each containing four sporozoites. Note: *I. hominis* oocysts are usually mature when passed by the host.

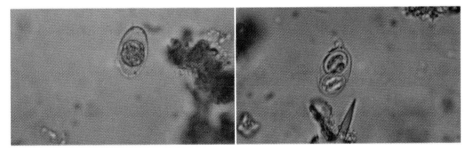

Figure 83. *Isospora belli* immature oocyst, unstained wet fecal preparation, X600. Criteria: Shape ellipsoidal; hyaline; single zygote. Note: *I. belli* oocysts are usually in this immature developmental stage when passed by the host.

Figure 84. *Isospora belli* mature oocyst, unstained wet fecal preparation, X600. Criteria: Shape ellipsoidal; hyaline; two sporocysts each containing four sporozoites. Note: *I. belli* oocysts are not passed in the mature stage of development. This oocyst was obtained from among those that had been aerated in a solution of 2 percent potassium dichromate to induce sporulation.

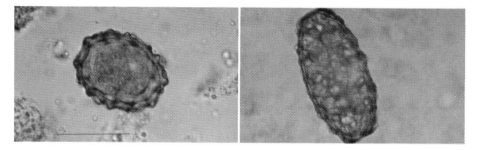

Figure 85. *Ascaris lumbricoides* fertilized egg, unstained wet fecal preparation, X400. Criteria: Shape usually ovoidal; brown; pronounced outer corticated membrane; large, round, unsegmented embryo.

Figure 86. *Ascaris lumbricoides* unfertilized egg, unstained wet fecal preparation, X400. Criteria: Shape usually oval-elongate; brown; pronounced outer corticated membrane; thin shell membrane; contents globular.

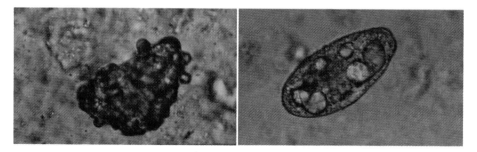

Figure 87. *Ascaris lumbricoides* unfertilized egg, unstained wet fecal preparation, X400. Criteria: Shape triangular; brown; pronounced outer corticated membrane; thin shell membrane; contents globular. Note: Unfertilized eggs of *A. lumbricoides* often assume various shapes.

Figure 88. *Ascaris lumbricoides* unfertilized egg, unstained wet fecal preparation, X400. Criteria: Shape usually oval-elongate; decorticated; thin shell membrane; contents globular. Note: This egg and the one illustrated in Figure 87 are often mistaken for plant cells.

26

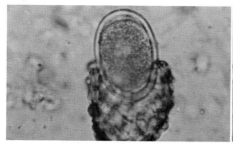 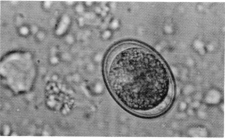

Figure 89. *Ascaris lumbricoides* fertilized egg, unstained wet fecal preparation, X400. Criteria: Shape usually ovoidal; brown outer corticated membrane, colorless thick shell membrane; large, round, unsegmented embryo. Note: The separation from the outer corticated membrane probably occurred during centrifugation of the fecal specimen from which this egg was obtained.

Figure 90. *Ascaris lumbricoides* fertilized egg, unstained wet fecal preparation, X400. Criteria: Shape usually ovoidal; decorticated; colorless thick shell membrane; large, round, unsegmented embryo.

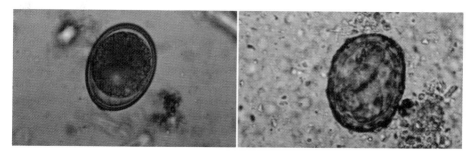

Figure 91. *Ascaris lumbricoides* fertilized egg, iodine stained wet fecal preparation, X400. Criteria: Shape usually ovoidal; decorticated; thick shell membrane; large, round, unsegmented embryo.

Figure 92. *Ascaris lumbricoides* fully embryonated egg, unstained wet fecal preparation, X400. Criteria: Shape usually ovoidal; brown outer corticated membrane. Note: The fecal specimen from which this egg was recovered was incubated at room temperature for several days allowing the embryo to develop to the larval form.

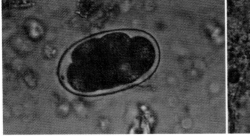 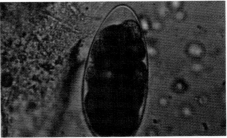

Figure 93. Hookworm egg, unstained wet fecal preparation, X400. Criteria: Shape ovoidal; rounded ends; hyaline; thin shell membrane; segmented embryo, usually 2 to 8 cells.

Figure 94. *Trichostrongylus* spp. egg, unstained wet fecal preparation, X400. Criteria: Shape oval-elongate; one or both ends pointed; hyaline; thin shell membrane; segmented embryo, usually 8 or more cells. Note: This egg is much larger than a hookworm egg. See Figure 93.

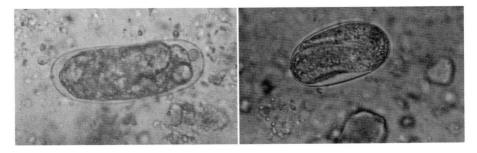

Figure 95. *Heterodera marioni* egg, unstained wet fecal preparation, X400. Criteria: Shape ellipsoidal; rounded ends; one side slightly indented; hyaline; thin shell membrane; polar globules usually present; embryo usually in early stages of cleavage. Note: *H. marioni* is a plant parasite. Its eggs may be found in fecal specimens from persons who have ingested root type vegetables.

Figure 96. Hookworm egg, unstained wet fecal preparation, X400. Criteria: Shape ovoidal; rounded ends; hyaline, thin shell membrane. Note: A larva is often seen within a hookworm egg obtained from a fecal specimen that is several hours old.

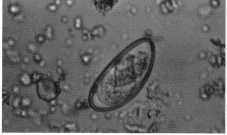 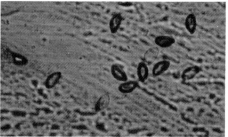

Figure 97. *Enterobius vermicularis* egg, unstained wet fecal preparation, X400. Criteria: Shape ovoidal; one side flattened; hyaline; thick shell membrane; usually a fully developed larva within the egg.

Figure 98. *Enterobius vermicularis* eggs, cellulose tape preparation, X100. Criteria: Shapes ovoidal and flat on one side; hyaline. Note: When examining this type of a preparation, be certain not to mistake air bubbles for pinworm eggs.

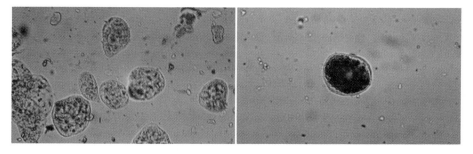

Figure 99. Plant cells, unstained wet fecal preparation, X100. Criteria: Shapes irregular; usually various sizes; contents globular. Note: An inexperienced examiner may mistake these cells for worm eggs.

Figure 100. Plant cell, iodine stained wet fecal preparation, X100. Criteria: Shape irregular; contents brown and globular.

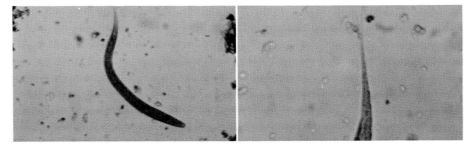

Figure 101. Hookworm rhabditiform larva, iodine stained wet fecal preparation, X150. Criteria: Long, sharp, needle-like tail.

Figure 102. Hookworm rhabditiform larva, iodine stained wet fecal preparation, X600. Criteria: Long, slender, needle-like extension of the cuticula. Note: This is a greater magnification of the larva's tail illustrated in Figure 101.

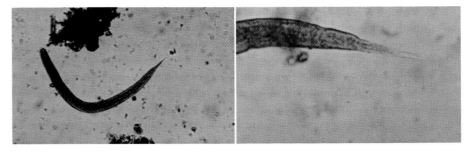

Figure 103. *Strongyloides stercoralis* rhabditiform larva, iodine stained wet fecal preparation, X150. Criterion: Tail tapers to a fine point. Note: The tail is not as long as that of hookworm. See Figure 101.

Figure 104. *Strongyloides stercoralis* rhabditiform larva, iodine stained wet fecal preparation, X600. Criterion: Tail tapers to a fine point. Note: This is a greater magnification of the larva's tail illustrated in Figure 103. Its tail differs from that of hookworm in that it is not as long, slender and needle-like. See Figure 102.

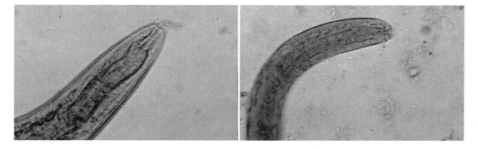

Figure 105. Hookworm rhabditiform larva, iodine stained wet fecal preparation, X600. Criterion: Long buccal groove (longer than the head is wide).

Figure 106. *Strongyloides stercoralis* rhabditiform larva, iodine stained wet fecal preparation, X600. Criterion: Short buccal groove (shorter than the head is wide).

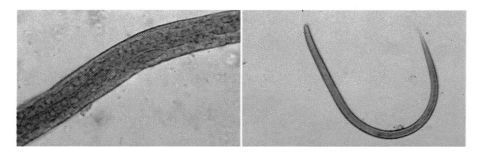

Figure 107. *Strongyloides stercoralis* rhabditiform larva, iodine stained wet fecal preparation, X600. Criterion: Large genital primordium. Note: The genital primordium of a hookworm larva is so small that it usually is indistiguishable from other internal anatomical features.

Figure 108. *Strongyloides stercoralis* filariform larva, iodine stained wet fecal preparation, X150. Criteria: Body long and slender. Note: Compare this larva with the ones illustrated in Figures 101 and 103.

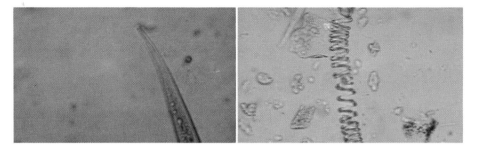

Figure 109. *Strongyloides stercoralis* filariform larva, iodine stained wet fecal preparation, X600. Criterion: Notched tail. Note: This is a greater magnification of the larva's tail illustrated in Figure 108.

Figure 110. Vegetable spiral, unstained wet fecal preparation, X400. Criterion: Bedspring-shaped.

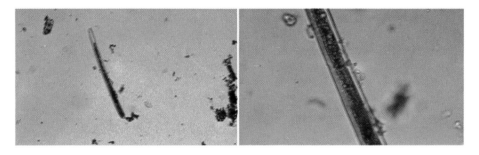

Figure 111. Plant fiber, iodine stained wet fecal preparation, X100. Note: An inexperienced examiner may superficially mistake this fiber for a worm larva.

Figure 112. Plant fiber, iodine stained wet fecal preparation, X400. Criteria: Thick wall; disorganized internal structure. Note: This is a greater magnification of the same plant fiber illustrated in Figure 111.

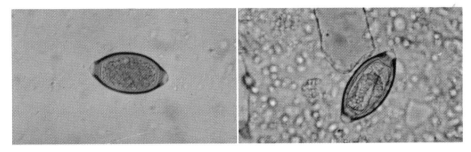

Figure 113. *Trichuris trichiura* egg, unstained wet fecal preparation, X400. Criteria: Barrel-shaped; brown; polar mucoid plugs; double, thick shell membrane; unsegmented embryo usually fills the entire egg.

Figure 114. *Trichuris trichiura* fully embryonated egg, unstained wet fecal preparation, X400. Criteria: Barrel-shaped; brown; polar mucoid plugs; double, thick shell membrane. Note: The fecal specimen from which this egg was recovered was incubated at room temperature for several days allowing the embryo to develop to the larval form.

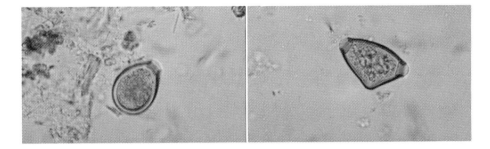

Figure 115. *Trichuris trichiura* atypical egg, unstained wet fecal preparation, X400. Criteria: Brown; mucoid plug; double thick shell membrane; unsegmented embryo usually fills the entire egg. Note: This abnormally formed egg was recovered from a patient's fecal specimen who was undergoing treatment for trichuriasis.

Figure 116. *Trichuris trichiura* atypical egg, unstained wet fecal preparation, X400. Criteria: Brown; mucoid plugs; double thick shell membrane. Note: This abnormally formed egg was also recovered from the same patient's fecal specimen who was undergoing treatment for trichuriasis. See Figure 115.

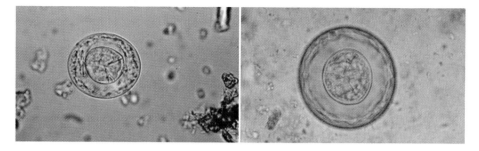

Figure 117. *Hymenolepis nana* egg, unstained wet fecal preparation, X400.
Criteria: Shape spherical to ovoidal; hyaline; thin shell membrane; embryo with
prominent hooklets; thread-like polar fila-
ments.

Figure 118. *Hymenolepis diminuta* egg,
unstained wet fecal preparation, X400.
Criteria: Shape spherical; yellowish-
brown; shell membrane thickened; embryo with prominent hooklets.

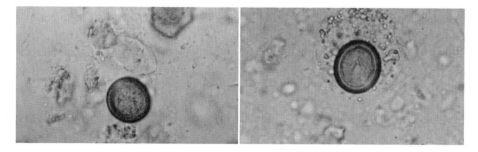

Figure 119. *Taenia* spp. egg, unstained
wet fecal preparation, X400. Criteria:
Shape spherical; brown; thick shell with
striations; embryo with prominent hooklets.

Figure 120. *Taenia* spp. egg enclosed in
its embryonic membrane, unstained wet
fecal preparation, X400. Criteria: Hyaline
embryonic membrane; egg spherical;
brown; thick shell with striations; embryo
with prominent hooklets.

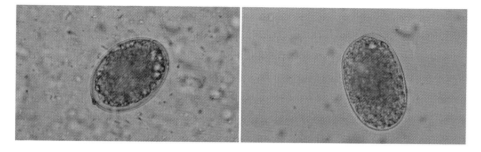

Figure 121. *Diphyllobothrium latum* egg, unstained wet fecal preparation, X400. Criteria: Shape ovoidal; yellowish; shell membrane thickened; conspicuous operculum; small abopercular button; contents globular.

Figure 122. Hookworm egg, unstained wet fecal preparation, X400. Criteria: Shape ovoidal; rounded ends; hyaline; thin shell membrane; contents globular. Note: An unsegmented hookworm egg is often mistaken for a *D. latum* egg. Notice the thinness of the shell and the absence of an operculum. See Figure 121.

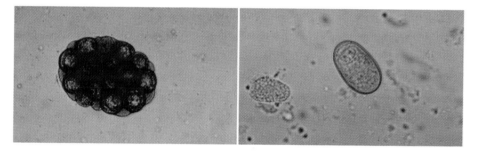

Figure 123. *Dipylidium caninum* egg packet, unstained wet fecal preparation, X150. Criteria: Large size; several eggs enclosed within a capsule.

Figure 124. *Dicrocoelium dendriticum* egg, unstained wet fecal preparation, X400. Criteria: Shape ovoidal; brown; thick shell membrane; operculate; mature miracidium within the egg.

35

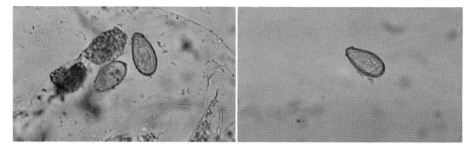

Figure 125. *Clonorchis sinensis* eggs, unstained wet fecal preparation, X400. Criteria: Pear-shaped; brownish-yellow; thick shell membrane; conspicuous operculum with prominent shoulders; usually a comma-shaped abopercular protuberance; mature miracidium within the egg.

Figure 126. *Clonorchis sinensis* egg, unstained wet fecal preparation, X400. Criteria: Pear-shaped; brownish-yellow; thick shell membrane; conspicuous operculum with prominent shoulders; frequently a small abopercular button; mature miracidium within the egg. Note: The morphology of the abopercular protuberance often varies. See Figure 125.

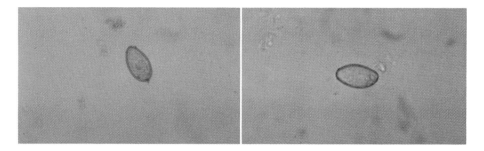

Figure 127. *Opisthorchis viverrini* egg, unstained wet fecal preparation, X400. Criteria: Pear-shaped; brownish-yellow; thick shell membrane; conspicuous operculum with prominent shoulders; a comma-shaped or button-like abopercular protuberance; mature miracidium within the egg. Note: This egg is smaller than that of *C. sinensis*. See Figures 125 and 126.

Figure 128. *Metagonimus yokogawai* egg, unstained wet fecal preparation, X400. Criteria: Shape ovoidal; brownish-yellow; thick shell membrane; operculum without prominent shoulders; usually a small abopercular button; mature miracidium within the egg.

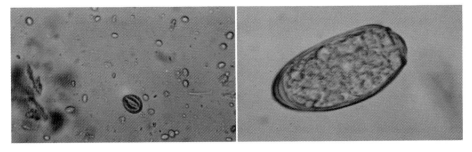

Figure 129. Pollen grain, unstained wet fecal preparation, X400. Note: Depending on geographic location and season of the year, different kinds of pollen grains are often recovered in fecal specimens. They must not be mistaken for worm eggs.

Figure 130. *Paragonimus westermani* egg, unstained wet fecal preparation, X400. Criteria: Shape ovoidal; brown; thick shell membrane; prominent operculum located at the broader anterior end; contents globular.

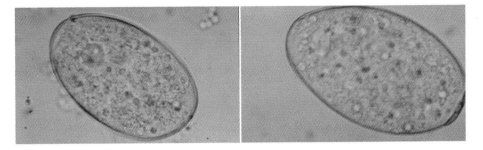

Figure 131. *Fasciola hepatica* egg, unstained wet fecal preparation, X400. Criteria: Shape ovoidal; very large size; yellowish-brown; large operculum; contents globular.

Figure 132. *Fasciolopsis buski* egg, unstained wet fecal preparation, X400. Criteria: Shape ovoidal; very large size; yellowish-brown; large operculum; contents globular. Note: This egg is usually larger and its operculum smaller than that of an egg of *F. hepatica*. See Figure 131.

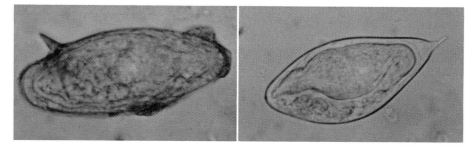

Figure 133. *Schistosoma mansoni* egg, unstained wet fecal preparation, X400. Criteria: Shape oval-elongate; large size; yellowish-brown; prominent lateral spine; non-operculate; usually a mature miracidium within the egg.

Figure 134. *Schistosoma haematobium*, unstained wet urine preparation, X400. Criteria: Shape oval-elongate; large size; yellowish; prominent terminal spine; non-operculate; usually a mature miracidium within the egg. Note: This egg is recovered in urine, rarely in feces.

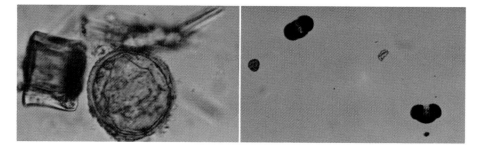

Figure 135. *Schistosoma japonicum*, unstained wet fecal preparation, X400. Criteria: Shape usually ovoidal, frequently spherical; brown; non-operculate; usually a mature miracidium within the egg. Note: A small lateral button or spine may occasionally be observed on the egg shell, but it is often so inconspicuous that it is difficult to see.

Figure 136. Pine pollen, unstained wet fecal preparation, X100. Criterion: Mickey mouse hat.

REFERENCES

1. Belding, D. L.: Textbook of Parasitology, 3rd ed. New York, Appleton-Century-Crofts, 1965.
2. Brooke, M. M.: Intestinal Protozoa. In Blair, J. E., Lennette, E. H. and Truant, J. P. (Ed.): Manual of Clinical Microbiology. Bethesda, American Society for Microbiology, 1970.
3. Faust, E. C., Russell, P. F. and Jung, R. C.: Craig and Faust's Clinical Parasitology, 8th ed. Philadelphia, Lea and Febiger, 1970.
4. Hunter, G. W., III, Frye, W. W. and Swartzwelder, J. C.: A Manual of Tropical Medicine, 4th ed. Philadelphia and London, Saunders, 1966.
5. Markell, E. K. and Voge, M.: Medical Parasitology, 3rd ed. Philadelphia, London, Toronto, Saunders, 1971.
6. Spencer, F. M. and Monroe, L. S.: The Color Atlas of Intestinal Parasites. Springfield, Thomas, 1961.
7. Swartzwelder, J. C., Miller, J. H., Abadie, S. H. and Warren, L. G.: Helminths. In Blair, J. E., Lennette, E. H. and Truant, J. P. (Ed.): Manual of Clinical Microbiology. Bethesda, American Society for Microbiology, 1970.

INDEX

A

Amebas, 5-14, 18-23
Ancylostoma duodenale (see Hookworm)
Ascaris lumbricoides, 26, 27
  decorticated eggs, 26, 27
  fertilized eggs, 26, 27
  unfertilized eggs, 26, 27

B

Balantidium coli, 24
Blastocystis hominis, 17
Blood flukes (*see* Schistosomes)
Broad tapeworm (*see Diphyllobothrium latum)*

C

Cestodes, 34, 35
Charcot-Leyden crystals, 17
Chilomastix mesnili, 15, 16, 24
  cysts, 15, 24
  trophozoites, 16
Chinese liver fluke (*see Clonorchis sinensis*)
Ciliate (*see Balantidium coli*)
Clonorchis sinensis, 36
Coccidia, 25

D

Dicrocoelium dendriticum, 35
Dientamoeba fragilis, 8
Diphyllobothrium latum, 35
Dipylidium caninum, 35
Dog tapeworm (*see Dipylidium caninum*)
Dwarf tapeworm (*see Hymenolepis nana*)

E

Endolimax nana, 7, 8, 13, 14, 20
  cysts, 13, 14, 20
  trophozoites, 7, 8
Entamoeba coli, 5, 6, 11-13, 18, 21-23
  cysts, 11-13, 18, 21-23
    immature, 11, 18, 21-23
    mature, 12, 13, 22
  trophozoites, 5, 6
Entamoeba hartmanni, 6, 8, 13, 14, 19, 20
  cysts, 13, 14, 19, 20
    immature, 13, 19
    mature, 14, 20
  trophozoites, 6, 8
Entamoeba histolytica, 5, 6, 9, 10, 12, 18, 19, 21-23
  cysts, 9, 10, 12, 18, 19, 21-23
    immature, 9, 10, 18, 19, 21
    mature, 12, 22, 23
  trophozoites, 5, 6
Enterobius vermicularis, 29

F

Fasciola hepatica, 37
Fasciolopsis buski, 37
Fish tapeworm (*see Diphyllobothrium latum*)
Flagellates, 15, 16, 24
Flukes (*see* Trematodes)

G

Giardia lamblia, 15, 24
  cysts, 15, 24
  trophozoites, 15, 24

H

Heterodera marioni, 28

41